10 Essential Herbs for Lifelong Health

Barbara Heller, M.S.W.

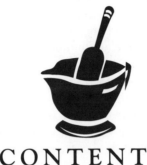

D1706502

CONTENTS

Why Use Herbs?

Throughout the ages, plants have served a multitude of uses for human survival. Ethnobotany, the study of plant lore and agricultural customs, has provided us with rich evidence of the ways different cultures have traditionally used plants to feed and nourish, house and clothe, inform and educate, and treat and heal bodies and spirits.

These days, people increasingly are using natural remedies for health and healing. Polls show that more than 30 percent of the U.S. population has recently used one of the many alternative therapies, which include herbal medicine, chiropractic, acupuncture, and massage. In fact, North American consumers spend more than $3.2 billion a year on herbal remedies, and that number continues to increase. Many people are turning away from synthetic medications, both over-the-counter and prescription. They want to use more natural substances — and scientific research supports claims of the reliability, safety, and effectiveness of many herbal treatments (when they are used properly, of course).

The Proof

As another sign of the changing times, the large and somewhat daunting *Physician's Desk Reference (PDR)* — a standard reference book found in most medical offices that describes all available chemical prescription drugs — has recently issued both an herbal medicine edition and a family guide to natural remedies.

Choosing and Using Natural Remedies

There are lots of wonderful ways to use herbs. Most herbalists suggest using the fresh- or dried-plant formulations, preferably from herbs grown locally and organically. However, for many of us that's not possible, and it's more convenient to purchase commercial preparations. Prepackaged herbal teas and capsules are now found in many supermarkets and pharmacies. Specialty stores carry loose herbs as well as herbal tinctures and infused oils. You can also use store-bought or homemade herbal skin salves, bath salts, and toiletries.

Herbal Teas

Mmmmm . . . an evening cup of chamomile tea, perhaps after a warm bath, can help you to slow down and ease you to sleep. A cup of peppermint tea can soothe a stomachache, while a mug of warming ginger can lessen nausea. Mild herbal teas — prepared as infusions or decoctions — can be both aromatic and soothing, and a tea blend made from a variety of plants can impart many healing qualities. Many herbal teas are noncaffeinated, unlike the common green and black teas, which contain caffeine and tannin and are stimulating. Green and black teas, however, also have health benefits in the areas of reducing cancer risk, supporting the cardiovascular system, and normalizing intestinal flora.

Herbal tea blends are manufactured by many companies; boxes of blended tea bags are readily available. Due to governmental regulations, companies cannot make health claims about their products. But their evocative names, like Tranquil-A-Tea, Mama Bear's Echinacea Cold Care, Sleepy-Time, and Heart's Ease, often provide clues to the conditions they are meant to treat.

MAKING AN HERBAL INFUSION

When making a tea from leaves, flowers, berries, or seeds, you'll want to infuse them. These ingredients easily release their essential oils when they're steeped in hot water — and they easily lose their value when they're simmered. For simple enjoyment, many people make mild infusions from some of the more pleasant-tasting herbs, such as peppermint and raspberry leaf. For medicinal purposes, however, the tea must be made stronger — i.e., steeped longer — and it may not always taste pleasant.

1   **cup (237 ml) boiling water**
1   **teaspoon (5 ml) dried herb** or **1 tablespoon (15 ml) fresh herb** or **a prepackaged tea bag**

Bring the water to a boil. Place the herb or tea bag in a mug. Pour the water over the herb; cover. For a mild tea, let steep for about 5 minutes; for a stronger, more potent tea, steep for at least 20 minutes and up to several hours — even overnight. If you've used loose herb, strain before drinking.

MAKING AN HERBAL DECOCTION

A decoction is a tea made from plant roots or bark. Because these plant parts are tougher and more fibrous than leaves and flowers, they must be simmered in boiling water to extract their medicinal qualities.

1 **cup (237 ml) water**
1 **teaspoon (5 ml) dried herb** or 1 **tablespoon (15 ml) fresh herb**

Combine the water and herb in a pot; cover. Bring to a boil, reduce heat, and let simmer for 20 minutes.

You can, of course, make tea in large batches. Keep it refrigerated and reheat in a saucepan in small amounts to be served throughout the day.

Herb Use and Environmental Concerns

As the popular herbalist and author Susun Weed said, "Do not sacrifice planetary health for personal health." All of our health-care decisions have environmental implications; this is especially true when considering herbal remedies. Where were the plants grown and how were they obtained? Are the herbs organically grown? Is the plant endangered?

For many of us, this consideration may seem like a huge burden. Obviously, when we are feverish and feeling as if we are coming down with the flu, we want a helpful remedy right away. We don't want to stop and think about the environmental implications of our decision. Perhaps we can think about these larger concerns as we begin to learn about herbal remedies and start to stock our herbal medicine cabinets.

The overharvesting of wild plants to satisfy the commercial demand for herbal products is of valid concern to many naturalists. For example, stands of wild echinacea and ginseng have been depleted and negative changes are evident in the surrounding ecosystems where large amounts of the herbs have been picked. Some prepared products state the kinds of plants that were used in processing. It is ecologically prudent to purchase organically grown, as opposed to "wildcrafted" products. It is our responsibility to promote respect for the environment and ethical plant harvesting.

Herbal Tinctures

When a more potent herbal remedy is needed, you can take a liquid herbal formula. Dr. Andrew Weil recommends tinctures as one of your most reliable and most effective purchases. A tincture is an herbal preparation that combines a specific herb with an agent to draw out and preserve its medicinal qualities. An alcohol base is common because alcohol can extract and preserve the most useful plant constituents. Glycerin-based tinctures are good alternatives for children and those sensitive to alcohol.

Tinctures are convenient and have a long shelf life. In addition, they are easily portable and make a wonderful addition to a traveler's medical kit.

MAKING AN HERBAL TINCTURE

To tincture, you must first process — mince fresh herbs or powder dried herbs — to release the essential oils.

For fresh herbs:
- 1   **part herb, coarsely chopped or minced**
- 2   **parts vodka, brandy, apple cider vinegar, or glycerin**

For dried herbs:
- 1   **part herb, powdered**
- 3   **parts vodka, brandy, apple cider vinegar, or glycerin**

1. Put the processed herbs in a widemouthed jar. The herbs should make up about a quarter of the total volume. Cover the herbs with the liquid. Stir well, then seal the jar tightly and place in a dark location. Shake the jar once a day for 2 to 4 weeks.

2. Strain the liquid and decant into smaller, dark glass bottles. Store tinctures at room temperature in a dark, cool place.

Note: When tincturing with vinegar, cover the top of the jar with plastic wrap before putting on the lid. Otherwise, fumes from the vinegar will corrode the lid, making it difficult to open.

Herbal Oils and Salves

Herbal oils and salves provide soothing external comfort for many muscle aches, skin irritations, bruises, and minor burns. They can be made at home or purchased from herb shops and most health-food stores.

MAKING AN INFUSED OIL

2–3   **ounces (56–85 g) dried or fresh-wilted herb**
1   **pint (473 ml) olive oil**

1. Put the herb in a jar and add the oil, making sure there are 2 to 3 inches (5–7.5 cm) of oil on top of the herb.

2. Cover the jar with four layers of cheesecloth and secure with a rubber band or the outer ring of the jar lid. Place the jar in a warm, dry spot (such as a sunny window-sill or on top of a water heater) for 2 weeks.

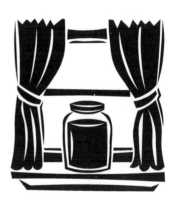

3. Strain and press the oil from the herbs. Store in an airtight container (preferably dark glass) in a cool, dark location. The oil will keep for 3 to 6 months.

MAKING A SALVE

1   **cup (237 ml) infused oil**
¼   **cup (59 ml) grated beeswax**

1. Combine the oil and the beeswax in the top of a double boiler. Heat until the beeswax is melted, stirring thoroughly. Remove from heat.

2. To test the consistency of the salve, put a spoonful of the mixture in the refrigerator for a minute or two. If it's too hard, add more oil. If it doesn't harden, add a bit more bees-wax. Store salve in tightly sealed glass containers. When refrigerated, it should keep for up to a year.

Essential Oils

Essential oils are concentrated essences of the naturally occurring oils in plants and flowers. They are primarily used in perfumes and aromatherapy. Essential oils are absorbed by our bodies both through our skin and by smell. Like herbs, they have unique healing qualities. The oils are extracted from the plants by a pressure method or by steam distillation. These are large-scale commercial operations and are not appropriate projects for do-it-yourselfers — it takes hundreds or even thousands of pounds of a plant to make just one ounce of essential oil.

Do not confuse essential oils with their synthetic counterparts, which are often sold for hobby and craft purposes. The synthetic oils do not provide the healing qualities of the pure essences. True essential oils vary greatly in price from each other, depending on the rarity and density of the plant and the country in which it was processed. For example, oils made from lemons and lavender are relatively reasonable in price, while those made from roses are so expensive that people sometimes purchase them by the drop rather than by the ounce!

Essential Oil Caution

Enjoy essential oils in external applications — massage oils, herbal bath mixtures, and compresses. They are also good additions to homemade cleaning products. Do not take them internally, however, unless directed to do so by a qualified healthcare professional. In addition, use just the amount specified in a recipe — if three drops are called for, ten drops are not necessarily better and can, in fact, be harmful.

Herbal Steams and Compresses

Have a cold? Feeling congested? An over-the-counter antihistamine can help, but it may cause drowsiness, dry mouth, constipation, or other side effects. Perhaps you have a headache and aspirin upsets your stomach. If you want to try something milder, why not start with a steam or compress? Then follow it with a hot cup of herbal tea.

HERBAL STEAMS

A steam will greatly relieve stuffiness and other related cold symptoms. As a bonus, it can also help clear up skin problems.

A small handful of dried herbs
Boiling water

1. Place the herbs in a large nonplastic bowl. Pour in the boiling water, filling the bowl no more than three-quarters full.

2. "Tent" a towel over your head and the bowl and savor the wafting scents. Take care not to burn yourself: Don't bend too low, and make sure that the bowl is sitting securely on the surface.

Step 2

To make a compress: Combine the herb with boiling water in a bowl. Let the liquid cool until you can touch it, then saturate a clean cloth with the warm, aromatic water. Carefully squeeze out the excess and apply the cloth to the affected area. Compresses can be especially comforting to headache sufferers.

Herbal Baths

Aromatic herbal baths are wonderfully soothing and health promoting. Some aromas, such as lavender and chamomile, are relaxing; others, like peppermint, are stimulating. Herbal baths are especially helpful for insomnia and stress-related ailments as well as an adjunct for treating colds and fevers.

Bath salts are a great way to incorporate herbs into the bath. Although ready-made bath salts can be purchased, you can make your own by mixing equal parts of sea salt, Epsom salts, and baking soda. Then add a fragrant essential oil or a mixture of oils — 10 to 15 drops per cup of the salt mixture. Pour the salts into the bath as the tub is filling; as they dissolve, they emit a lovely aroma.

Bath bags are another convenient way to immerse yourself in herbal pleasure. Simply place a handful of herbs in the middle of a clean, square cloth and tie it closed. It's like

> ### Caution
> Pregnant women should not take herbal baths except under the advice of a medical practitioner.

making a large tea bag to brew in a very large "teapot" — your bathtub. Hang the sachet from the bathtub faucet and let the water run through the herbs.

Ten Essential Herbs

In today's marketplace, there are many "popular" herbs renowned for their medicinal qualities. The ten herbs discussed here are among those that are particularly well known. Because they are also easy to use, widely available, and recommended for treating an amazingly wide range of ailments, they are well suited for presenting a basic overview and introduction to the ways in which herbs can help create health, happiness, and harmony in your life.

10 Herbs at a Glance

Although each herb can be used in many different ways, here is a quick summary of their primary uses.

Herb	Primary Use
Calendula	Applied externally in the form of salves and ointments for treating skin irritations
Chamomile	Taken as a tea that calms and relaxes; also good for stomachaches
Echinacea	Taken in tincture or capsule form to boost the immune system and help fight off colds and flu
Garlic	Eaten or applied raw as an antibacterial and antiviral and for cardiovascular benefits; eaten cooked, retains only cardiovascular benefits.
Ginger	Eaten raw or in capsule form to combat motion sickness, nausea, indigestion, and inflammation
Lavender	The herb and essential oil are used in baths and compresses to treat insomnia, headaches, and burns
Lemon balm	Taken as a tea that acts to calm, soothe, and uplift
Peppermint	Taken as a tea that soothes stomachaches and headaches and eases symptoms of colds and flu
St.-John's-wort	Taken as a tea or in tincture or capsule form to treat mild to moderate depression or anxiety
Valerian	Taken in tincture or capsule form to relieve anxiety and nervous tension

Calendula (*Calendula officinalis*)

Calendula is a versatile plant that has been used for its medicinal, culinary, and cosmetic qualities and as a dye. Used in salves and ointments, calendula is a potent skin healer. Its primary culinary use is as an edible flower garnish. The brightly colored and mildly flavored calendula flower petals, fresh or dried, can be added to salads, soups, and muffins. Dried and ground, calendula can be substituted for the more expensive saffron.

Herbal History

The ancient Romans grew calendula primarily for its ornamental qualities and also as a remedy for scorpion bites. In medieval households, calendula blossoms were often used in soups, salads, puddings, and wine. Although used in folk medicine, calendula was never considered a major medicinal herb. Instead, it was most revered for its magical attributes. Calendula potions were thought to enable those who drank them to see fairies or decide between suitors.

Calendula in the Garden

Also known as pot marigold, calendula is an easy-to-grow, long-blooming annual. A sun-loving plant, it is said that one can predict the weather by its blossoms: If they do not open in the early morning, it is a forecast for rain. The plant usually grows 6 to 18 inches (15–45 cm) tall and blooms from June through October. Some of the newer varieties have stronger stems, growing to 30 inches (75 cm), and make lovely cut flowers. The centers of the flowers differ, some are light and others dark, which creates a beautiful contrast in the garden.

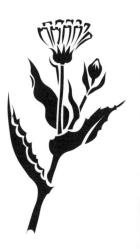

Health Benefits

With antibacterial, antifungal, antiviral, and immune-stimulating properties, calendula is perfectly designed for soothing and healing the skin. It is primarily used in external preparations for myriad skin conditions. Calendula soothes cuts, bruises, diaper rash, eczema, hemorrhoids, burns, and other mild or chronic conditions. Germany's Commission E recommends calendula to speed wound healing and treat skin inflammations.

Some herbalists also recommend calendula in mouthwashes to treat sores and gingivitis. Calendula tea or tincture can be used for heartburn relief and as a part of ulcer treatment because of its ability to lower stomach acid levels.

How to Use Calendula

A soothing calendula skin salve, store-bought or homemade, makes a great addition to a medicine kit. Diluted calendula tincture may be used externally for topical skin care or internally for acid stomach. A cooled brewed tea of calendula can be used as a wash for minor skin complaints. Dried and ground calendula makes a good base for a body powder when mixed with cornstarch. Many baby soaps and lotions contain calendula because of its mild, soothing properties.

SOOTHING CALENDULA SKIN SALVE

Use this salve to soothe and heal mild burns, bruises, cuts, and rashes.

1	cup (237 ml) calendula infused oil (see recipe on page 12)
2	ounces (56 g) beeswax, grated
4–10	drops lavender essential oil
1	200 IU vitamin E capsule

1. Combine the infused oil with the beeswax in the top of a double boiler. Heat gently until the beeswax has melted, stirring frequently. Remove from heat and allow to cool until you can touch it.

2. Add the lavender essential oil and the contents of the vitamin E capsule. Pour the mixture into small containers. The salve will solidify as it cools.

Note: The ratio of oil to beeswax is flexible and varies according to personal preference. To test the salve's consistency, put a spoonful of the beeswax mixture on a spoon and place in the freezer for 1 minute. If you want a firmer salve, add additional grated beeswax. For a softer salve, add more oil.

CALENDULA INFUSED OIL

You can use the infused oil by itself for topical healing of minor skin irritations.

2   parts extra-virgin olive oil
1   part dried calendula blossoms

1. Combine the olive oil and calendula blossoms in the top of a double boiler. Simmer gently for approximately 1 hour.

2. Strain the cooled mixture through a double layer of cheesecloth. Store in a cool, dark location, where it will keep for 3 to 6 months.

Safety and Cautions for Calendula

James Duke, botanist and author, points out that people who have hay fever may have an allergic reaction to this herb, especially if taken internally; he advises that a person stop taking it at the first sign of any itching or other discomfort. The *PDR for Herbal Medicines* states that there are no known health hazards or side effects when calendula is used in normal doses.

Chamomile *(Matricaria recutita)*

Chamomile's pretty white flowers with yellow centers make a lovely, mild, relaxing tea. (In the children's book, Peter Rabbit's mother served him a cup of chamomile after his escape from Mr. McGregor's garden.) Chamomile is good in baths for sleepless adults or fussy babies. Many herbalists also recommend this gentle herb as a colic remedy.

Chamomile in the Garden

German chamomile, a tall annual, has small, daisylike flowers with a wisp of apple scent. The flowers can be picked and dried to make tea. Both German chamomile and Roman chamomile *(Chamaemelum nobile),* a somewhat similar-looking perennial, are widely cultivated for commercial purposes.

Health Benefits

Chamomile has a relaxing effect on the nervous and digestive systems. In addition to being a sleep aid, chamomile has traditionally been used to treat stomachaches, ulcers, menstrual cramps, and arthritis. Chamomile tea is served to soothe heartburn, indigestion, and acid reflux.

Externally, chamomile has been used to heal wounds because of its anti-inflammatory properties. Compresses and baths made with infused flowers soothe irritated and inflamed skin. Several German studies have shown that applying a topical cream significantly reduced dermatitis. It is included on the list of herbs that the FDA deems "generally regarded as safe."

How to Use Chamomile

Serve chamomile as a soothing, sweetly scented tea. Although I often recommend infusing medicinal teas for a longer period of time, if you desire a mild, pleasant-tasting tea, don't steep chamomile for more than 10 minutes. It becomes bitter the longer it is steeped. You can brew it alone or in combination with other calming herbs, such as lemon balm. It is a major ingredient in many commercial tea blends, such as Celestial Seasonings Sleepytime tea. Extracts are also available.

Chamomile can also be used externally in baths or ointments, and its scent makes it a wonderful addition to potpourri, wreaths, and other aromatic herbal crafts.

 Herbal History

The ancient Egyptians used chamomile to treat the chills and fever of malaria. The Greeks and Romans used it to cure headaches and kidney, liver, and bladder disorders. Due to its pleasant scent, chamomile was used as a "strewing" herb, the medieval equivalent of a room freshener.

CALMING CHAMOMILE BATH BAGS

A warm bath with these fragrant sachets provides a gentle way to wind down from a stressful day. This recipe will make enough for eight baths.

2	**cups (473 ml) dried chamomile flowers**
1	**cup (237 ml) dried lavender flowers**
½	**cup (118 ml) dried hops flowers**
½	**cup (118 ml) dried passionflower**

Combine all ingredients. Place ½ cup (118 ml) of the mixture in the middle of a piece of permeable fabric and tie it closed. When running the bath, loop the tie over the faucet so that the water runs through the bag as the tub fills.

Safety and Cautions for Chamomile

As with all herbs, individual reactions may differ. Some people have an allergic reaction to chamomile, especially those who have hay fever and ragweed allergies, although the *PDR for Herbal Medicines* says that chamomile has a very weak potential for sensitization.

Echinacea (*Echinacea angustifolia, E. pallida,* or *E. purpurea*)

Also known as purple coneflower, echinacea makes a lovely addition to the garden. There are at least three echinacea species that have been used for their different medicinal properties. Although it is native to America, echinacea's medicinal effectiveness as a powerful immunity booster has been extensively studied in Germany.

Echinacea in the Garden

Purple coneflower is a tall, regal plant that adds wonderful end-of-the-season color to the perennial garden. It resembles a black-eyed Susan, but with purple rays.

Herbal History

Echinacea was a primary Native American healing herb. The Plains Indians used it to soothe bites from insects and snakes, clean wounds, and to treat the symptoms of flu, mumps, and smallpox. It was touted as a snakebite remedy in the late 1880s and became incorporated into conventional medical treatment. German studies of echinacea's medical uses began in the 1950s and continue today, all with positive results.

The root of an established plant, three to four years old, is the primary part used medicinally. The plant may be dug in the autumn and the root divided and then dried before use (Because of concerns about the overharvesting of echinacea, however, harvest only those plants you grow in your own garden.) Depending on the species of echinacea, however, commercial products may incorporate the whole dried plant.

Preserving the Medicine

Many naturalists are concerned that echinacea is being overharvested, possibly threatening its survival. If you purchase echinacea, be sure that it has been cultivated (preferrably using organic methods), not wildcrafted.

Health Benefits

Echinacea is an immune-system enhancer with antibacterial and antiviral properties. It boosts the white blood cells that fight infection, helps stave off colds and flu, and lessens the duration and severity of symptoms once they occur.

Recent European studies conclude that echinacea is most effective when taken at the first sign of symptoms. Supplemental vitamin C at this time may also help lessen the severity of the sickness.

Taken internally, this plant medicine can also help to treat middle ear, urinary tract, vaginal yeast, and other recurring infections. Applied as a topical liquid, echinacea acts as a topical anesthetic, raising the area's pain threshold, and promotes healing of all kinds of skin wounds, burns, sores, and eczema. Echinacea's effectiveness as a treatment for rheumatoid arthritis and cancer is also being studied.

Some people take echinacea as a daily supplement in an attempt to prevent illness. Most authorities discourage its daily use, which can create a tolerance of the herb and negate its positive effects.

How to Use Echinacea

Echinacea can be prepared in many forms: internally as a capsule, tablet, juice, tincture, or tea and externally in liquid form (juice, diluted tincture, or cooled tea) as a base for a poultice or skin wash. For medicinal purposes, most herbal practitioners recommend the tincture form; the tea is generally not strong enough. The usual dose is 1 dropperful of the tincture up to four times a day. Capsules of the freeze-dried extract are also a good choice for a potent dose. Follow the directions on the individual product label.

It is common for the tincture to create a tingling sensation on the tongue when ingested. This reaction is harmless — and some say it's a sure sign of the echinacea's potency.

ECHINACEA-ROOT TEA

Start drinking this tea at the first sign of a cold or flu. You'll know it's potent when your tongue feels a bit tingly after downing a mug.

- 1 **teaspoon (5 ml) dried echinacea root, or 1 tablespoon (15 ml) fresh**
- 1 **cup (237 ml) water**
- **Honey (optional)**

Combine the echinacea and water in a saucepan. Bring to a boil, cover, and let simmer for 20 to 30 minutes. Remove from heat and strain. Sweeten with honey, if desired, and drink.

Safety and Cautions for Echinacea

Echinacea use may cause mild digestive side effects; no major side effects have been reported at recommended doses. Those allergic to flowers in the Daisy family may experience an allergic reaction and, if so, should discontinue use.

Echinacea may worsen the symptoms of autoimmune illnesses, including lupus, multiple sclerosis, and rheumatoid arthritis. People with AIDS are also cautioned against using this herb.

Garlic (*Allium sativum*)

Garlic, also called the stinking rose, is a culinary and medicinal wonder. A member of the onion family, this pungent bulb has been revered for eons as a natural remedy. As a popular food, garlic has inspired festivals, monocrop farms, and a multitude of cookbooks and gardening books.

Garlic in the Garden

Garlic is a compound bulb made up of 4 to 15 cloves encased in a papery sheath. Plant garlic in the fall for the next summer's harvest or in the spring for fall harvest. In spring and summer, cut the flowers from the plant to encourage additional bulb growth. To prolong their shelf life, cure the bulbs by letting them sit in sun for 3 to 5 days, which will toughen their outer papery sheaths for winter storage.

Health Benefits

Garlic's many therapeutic qualities include decreasing cardiovascular risk by lowering overall cholesterol levels, thinning the blood, reducing high blood pressure, and increasing circulation. Studies have shown that eating just one garlic clove a day reduced cholesterol in test subjects by 9 percent, which is equivalent to an 18 percent decrease in heart attack risk.

Garlic is purported to have antibacterial, antibiotic, antifungal, and antiviral properties. So even if you don't abide by the old folk custom of wearing garlic around the neck, eating garlic will enhance the immune system, lessen the risk of getting sick, decrease cold and flu symptoms, and help to fight infection.

Garlic may also be an important addition to a cancer-preventing lifestyle. Studies show that among people who eat a garlic-rich diet, there are 30 percent fewer cases of colon cancer and 50 percent fewer stomach cancers than in those who eat little of this powerful herb. Garlic has also proved helpful in preliminary studies with AIDS patients.

Herbal History

Evidence of garlic use dates back to a 3000 B.C. Sumerian cuneiform tablet. The Greeks fed it to the pyramid builders to enhance their immunity, and the ancient Egyptians used it to treat a multitude of medical conditions. Before the advent of commercial antibiotics, garlic juice was the remedy of choice for infected wounds. During World War I, Army physicians used garlic to treat infections; it supplemented depleted antibiotic supplies during World War II, earning it the nickname "Russian penicillin."

The contemporary custom of hanging garlic braids in kitchens did not originate purely as a culinary convenience. Europeans hung braided garlic at their doorposts to keep out evil spirits.

How to Use Garlic

The most potent way to take garlic is to eat it raw. Some practitioners recommend eating one raw clove, finely chopped, three times a day, but this amount may cause reactions in the stomachs of those eating it as well as in the noses of those around them! In terms of its antibiotic properties, it is estimated that an average-size garlic clove is equivalent to one fifth of an average dose of penicillin.

Cooking garlic lessens its antibacterial and antiviral action — the heat inactivates allinase, one of garlic's healing enzymes. But one study showed that if peeled cloves are left to sit for 10 minutes before cooking, their healing compounds are not lost. Since there have been no definitive conclusions, more research is being done on the comparative value of cooked and raw garlic.

Even if cooking lessens garlic's healing qualities, it does not eliminate them. Cooked garlic still retains many of its active compounds. There are many tasty dishes that can help you incorporate garlic into your diet. In addition to various soups, entrées, and garlic bread, try salad dressings and vinegar spiked with garlic.

Garlic powder supplements are also available and are about as active as cooked garlic.

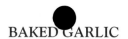

BAKED GARLIC

Baking a whole head of garlic softens its texture and taste. Individual cloves spread onto bread or baked potatoes are delicious, may help stave off a cold, and are a tasty way to include garlic's cancer-fighting and cholesterol-lowering qualities into your diet.

1   full head of garlic
Olive oil

1. Trim the top of the bulb slightly and cut the bottom so that it sits flat (do not peel off the papery sheath). Place on a baking dish and drizzle with the olive oil. Cover with aluminum foil. Bake at 350°F (175°C) for 1 hour, or until soft.

2. After the garlic has cooled, remove the foil. The roasted cloves will pop out easily when squeezed.

Safety and Cautions for Garlic

The *PDR for Herbal Medicines* reports that no health hazards or side effects are known for average levels of garlic consumption. For those with a sensitive stomach, however, ingesting garlic may cause gastrointestinal distress. Frequent contact has led to isolated cases of allergic skin reaction. Don't mix medicinal doses with hypertension medications or with blood thinners, including aspirin, taken for heart-attack prevention. Garlic's anticlotting action could cause problems for those with existing clotting disorders.

Ginger
(Zingiber officinalis)

What plant has been used to treat digestive difficulties for more than 25 centuries? What plant's root is used today for its powerful antinausea effects and as a treatment for rheumatoid arthritis? A container full of its ground essence probably sits on your spice shelf. The answer is ginger, the powerful attributes of which have been affirmed by historical, anecdotal, and scientific evidence.

Ginger in the Garden

Ginger is a tropical perennial. In the United States, this showy plant grows outdoors in Hawaii, Florida, and other states with hot steamy weather. Gingerroot, the rhizome or underground stem, is the plant part used medicinally. Limited quantities can be grown indoors from a cutting of a piece of store-bought ginger, although the older, toughened ginger most often available has a low propagation rate. The leaves grown from such a cutting are milder than the root, but may be used to enhance the flavor of cooked foods.

 Herbal History

Ginger has been used for centuries as a food and as a medication. We can thank the ancient Greeks for creating the original gingerbread treats. After dinner, as a digestive aid, the Greeks ate ginger wrapped in bread. Asian cultures have used ginger to prevent stomach upset and to relieve nausea.

Health Benefits

Ginger's primary use is as a remedy for motion sickness, nausea, and indigestion. Due to its anti-inflammatory qualities, it is also used to treat rheumatoid arthritis. A popular European remedy, ginger has been approved by Germany's Commission E. It is also listed as "generally regarded as safe" by the U.S. Food and Drug Administration.

Sailors and other travelers, take note: In multiple studies, ginger prevented motion sickness better and had fewer side effects than the leading over-the-counter motion sickness medication. Ginger's effectiveness has been proved in tests on Swedish seafaring naval cadets and on folks subjected to a tilting rotating chair and other simulated test situations intended to induce nausea. Ginger has also been hailed as an aid for postoperative nausea and to lessen the side effects of chemotherapy.

Ginger has a distinct advantage over conventional over-the-counter (OTC) antinausea medications. The OTCs act on the central nervous system and have a wide range of possible side effects, most notably fatigue. Ginger appears to avoid these adverse effects because it works on the digestive system instead of the central nervous system.

James Duke, former USDA botanist and author of *The Green Pharmacy*, lists more than 40 conditions that ginger is purported to help treat, including colds and flu, and cites it as a preventive against heart attack and stroke. Externally, ginger can be used in a massage oil to relieve lower back pain or in a wash to treat athlete's foot and other fungal infections.

How to Use Ginger

Pungent ginger can be enjoyed many ways. Fresh ginger is often available in the produce section of food markets; jars of dried powdered ginger are sold in the preserved herb and spice section. Ginger beverages are also popular. Ginger ale (the old-fashioned kind made without refined sugar, which negates ginger's actions) can soothe a stomachache. You can also make a tasty ginger tea. Try candied ginger, ginger cookies, and various spiced soups and dinner entrées as a way to increase your ginger intake.

Capsules of ground ginger are especially convenient during travel as a remedy for motion sickness. Take two 500 mg capsules (which contain about 1 gram of dried ginger) about a half hour before boarding. Take another dose if you become nauseated. Effects should last about 4 hours. A 1-inch-square (2.5 cm) piece of candied ginger or two cups of brewed tea can be substituted for a 500 mg capsule. Varro Tyler, a leading expert on herbs and plant-derived medicine, recommends a maximum daily dose of 4 grams.

GINGER TEA

This pungent remedy will help ease the symptoms of nausea or indigestion.

- 1   **cup (237 ml) water**
- 1   **teaspoon (5 ml) grated or powdered ginger**

1. Bring the water to a boil. Remove from heat, add the ginger, and cover. Let steep for at least 10 minutes.

2. Strain and enjoy!

Variations:

- Grate up to 1 tablespoon (15 ml) fresh ginger into a cup of brewed black or green tea.
- For a homemade ginger ale, mix a cup of strongly brewed ginger tea with carbonated water and lemon.

Safety and Cautions for Ginger

The prolific health author Jean Carper, in her book *Miracle Cures*, reassures us that "no human studies have reported any adverse effects from ginger, nor are there any cases of ginger toxicity on record in the medical literature."

People taking anticoagulants or who have bleeding problems should limit their use of ginger. Excessive ginger use may raise blood pressure and be detrimental to those with gallstones. Supervised use is recommended for those taking ginger to counteract the nausea of chemotherapy (if a person's platelet count is low, ginger may promote gastrointestinal bleeding).

Lavender (*Lavandula officinalis*)

The beauty of its deep color and its highly evocative scent have made lavender a favorite for many centuries. Wonderfully versatile, it has been used as an ornamental plant, in cosmetics and perfumes, and for its medicinal and culinary qualities.

Lavender in the Garden

Lavender is a beautiful and relatively easy-to-grow garden perennial. Its scented silvery foliage is complemented by long flower spikes of various purple hues. Check out local garden suppliers for the variety best suited for your climate and gardening zone. Lovely fields of lavender are cultivated in French provinces and the British countryside. Commercially, an acre of lavender yields 12 to 20 pounds of the essential oil. To dry your own garden lavender, pick the stalks just before the flowers open, tie in small bundles, and air-dry upside down.

Health Benefits

Lavender has a long-standing reputation for its medicinal attributes. It is used externally to help combat insomnia, nervousness, and headaches and to soothe wounds, burns, and skin irritations. It is purported to

Herbal History

Lavender is a Mediterranean plant that was cultivated in ancient times to make perfumes. Its name comes from the Latin *lavare*, which means "to wash," and it has scented many bathwaters over the ages. Lavender was used in the public bathhouses of Rome and as an ingredient in the Egyptian mummification process. It was a favorite of English royalty for their gardens, teas, and linens.

have antispasmodic, analgesic, antidepressant, and antiseptic qualities. It has been shown to reduce the size of breast cancer tumors in mice; current studies are investigating its possible cancer-fighting components.

How to Use Lavender

Use luscious lavender in the bath, as a soothing compress for the head and neck, or in a sleep pillow. A mild tea, for external or internal purposes, can be brewed from lavender flowers and leaves. Lavender essential oil, in dilution, is convenient to use in bath salts, in massage oils, and for application to insect bites and other skin irritations.

LAVENDER HEADACHE COMPRESS

This compress is wonderful for the relief of tension headaches.

½   cup (118 ml) dried lavender flowers (and leaves, if available)
2   cups (473 ml) boiling water

1. Put the lavender in a teapot or similar container. Pour water over the plant matter and steep, tightly covered, for 20 minutes.

2. Strain the tea into a bowl. Soak a clean cloth in the tea and gently wring it out. Drape this warm aromatic compress on the forehead and eyes or on the back of the neck.

Safety and Cautions for Lavender

There are no health hazards reported with the normal use of lavender, although isolated cases of contact dermatitis have been reported in sensitive people using products containing the essential oil.

Lemon Balm
(Melissa officinalis)

The luscious citrus taste and aroma of lemon balm are relaxing and good for stomachaches. Lemon balm is also called melissa, which comes from the Greek word for honeybee, a fitting name because the plant's fragrance has always attracted swarms. Use this versatile herb as a great-tasting and relaxing tea. It also makes a lovely culinary garnish for salads.

Lemon Balm in the Garden

Lemon balm is a low-growing tender perennial with deeply veined light green leaves and pink and white flowers. It grows up to 3 feet (90 cm) tall but may also spread low in the garden. Lemon balm can be grown from seed; it self-seeds so easily that some gardeners curse it as a weed. But even if it is a little wild, many think the wonderful scent makes up for the inconvenience.

Health Benefits

Lemon balm makes a great herbal remedy for insomnia. In studies using a combination extract of valerian and lemon balm, the effects were shown to be as powerful as pharmaceutical sleep medications. In

Herbal History

Historically, lemon balm has been used to treat headaches, menstrual cramps, wounds, nervousness, and anxiety. The Romans were said to have introduced this plant to the British Isles, where it became an important addition to the medicinal gardens of many monasteries. The Greeks used lemon balm to soothe those bitten by dogs and scorpions. Lemon balm was a sunny accompaniment for the American colonists; in fact, Thomas Jefferson grew the plant in his Monticello gardens.

addition to its mild tranquilizing effect, it has antibacterial and antiviral properties and relieves anxiety, menstrual cramps, and mild digestive problems.

How to Use Lemon Balm

Tea made from fresh or dried lemon balm is refreshing anytime. A tincture or extract is good for a stronger medicinal dose. The glycerin tincture maintains a wonderfully potent lemon flavor: a sure pick-me-up for the winter doldrums. Lemon balm's calming qualities are put to good use in bath bags and sleep pillows.

Harvesting Hints

Lemon balm must be gathered before the plant flowers, because after blooming the plant's essential-oil content drops dramatically. In addition, dried lemon balm has an extremely short shelf life — 2 to 3 months at best.

LOVELY LEMON-LAVENDER SLEEP PILLOW

To help ease away anxiety and sleeplessness, try a sleep pillow.

2   parts dried lemon balm leaves
1   part dried lavender flowers
1   part hops strobiles

Combine the herbs. Put the mixture in a small drawstring bag or sew into a flat pillow and place between your pillow and pillowcase.

Safety and Cautions for Lemon Balm

The *PDR for Herbal Medicines* reports that "no health hazards or side effects are known in conjunction with the proper administration of designated therapeutic dosages." However, Michael Castleman, author of *Healing Herbs*, cautions that because lemon balm can interfere with a thyroid-stimulating hormone, those who have a thyroid problem should consult a medical practitioner before using it.

Peppermint (Mentha x piperita)

Peppermint and its mint cousins are some of the most popular garden herbs. As a commercial additive, mint can make your mouth zing when used as flavoring for after-dinner mints, other candies, over-the-counter cough remedies, and dental products. The mints can be used for a variety of medicinal, culinary, cosmetic, and craft purposes.

Peppermint in the Garden

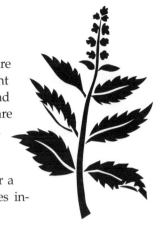

Mints are enthusiastic perennials with square stems. Growing about 2 feet tall, peppermint has sharply toothed, lance-shaped leaves and spreads by surface runners. Its flowers are small, pink to lavender, with four lobes. Mints can be invasive; to contain your peppermint, plant it in a pot in the ground.

Gardeners who are also cooks are in for a treat. The delicious medley of mint choices includes apple, chocolate, and pineapple.

Health Benefits

Peppermint's potent healing is derived from its aromatic oil, menthol. Menthol is antispasmodic, relaxing the muscles of the digestive tract. It's a wonderful digestive aid, mild enough to soothe children's stomachaches and excellent for adult indigestion and stomach upset. Studies show that menthol may also prevent stomach ulcers and stimulate bile secretion. Germany's Commission E has officially approved peppermint as an effective treatment for irritable bowel syndrome (IBS).

The decongestant action of peppermint also makes it a helpful adjunct in the treatment of many so-called winter ailments — the stuffiness and fever of colds and coughs as well as pneumonia. Peppermint chest rubs can ease the respiratory symptoms of colds.

 Herbal History

In the earliest medical texts of Egypt, mint was said to soothe stomachaches, although the mint suggested was probably a cousin to spearmint. Peppermint has similar effects but may be more powerful medicinally. It has certainly become more popular as a flavoring. The Greeks and Romans used mint to preserve milk as a curd and as a digestive aid. Hildegard von Bingen, the twelfth-century German abbess and herbalist, recommended mint as a treatment for gout and digestive problems. Both Native Americans and colonists used mints to treat respiratory conditions.

Safety and Cautions for Peppermint

There are no reports of problems caused by peppermint (the plant) in normal doses. Never ingest pure peppermint essential oil, which can be lethal. In rare cases, allergic reactions have been reported with external use of peppermint essential oil. Those with a tendency to have heartburn and gastroesophageal reflux should not ingest any form of peppermint; it irritates the condition. People with gallstones may experience digestive problems if they use peppermint products.

If you get peppermint oil in an eye or in an open wound, wash it out carefully with whole milk — the fat in the milk will bind with the oil. Do not use products with peppermint essential oil on the faces of young children because in rare cases, asthmalike symptoms and respiratory failure have been reported.

How to Use Peppermint

The most common and delicious way to enjoy peppermint is as a tea. A strong peppermint infusion makes a delicious morning pick-me-up, especially for those weaning themselves from coffee. Tinctures and capsules (enteric-coated ones are recommended for treating IBS) are also available. Diluted peppermint essential oil can be used in many external applications, including the treatment of tension headaches. Peppermint can also be added to the bath or used for compresses and steams.

Peppermint also seems to repel mice; put sprigs of dried peppermint near known rodent entrance holes to discourage mouse occupation. Try cotton balls sprinkled with peppermint essential oil as a deterrent to mice in the pantry.

BREATHE-EASY PEPPERMINT STEAM

Easy to prepare, a steam can help clear up the congestion of a cold.

- 2–4   cups (476–943 ml) boiling water
- ½   cup (118 ml) dried peppermint or 4–6 drops of peppermint essential oil

Place the dried peppermint in a metal or glass bowl and pour the boiling water over the herb, or add the essential oil to the water in the bowl. Tent a towel over your head and the bowl. Being careful not to burn yourself, breathe in the warm scent for a few minutes.

St.-John's-Wort
(Hypericum perforatum)

St.-John's-wort is a sunny plant that may brighten up dark dispositions. As a wild or cultivated plant, the vivid yellow flowers and green foliage produce a lovely dark red oil.

St.-John's-Wort in the Garden

St.-John's-wort stands 1 to 3 feet (30–91 cm) tall and bears bright yellow flowers. The leaves of this hardy perennial are perforated with many small holes, which can be seen when a leaf is held up to a light. When pinched, the leaves, flowers, and unopened buds all produce a red oil.

Health Benefits

St.-John's-wort is used internally for depression and anxiety and externally in the treatment of wounds, bruises, and first-degree burns.

St.-John's-wort's recently coined nickname, the Prozac of Plants, attests to its use as a highly effective and safe treatment for mild to moderate depression. It has been used extensively in Europe, and its popularity soared in the United States during the late 1990s. Studies show that St.-John's-wort is as effective as many

 ### Herbal History

St.-John's-wort was named by early Christians in honor of John the Baptist — the plant was said to bloom on his June birthday and bleed its red oil on the anniversary of the date the saint was beheaded. St.-John's-wort has been used as a cure for poisonous snake bites, in the treatment of malaria, and as a menstrual promoter. Both Native Americans and colonists used it to treat a variety of maladies, including wounds and skin problems.

prescription antidepressants, with a much lower rate of side effects. Many sufferers of Seasonal Affective Disorder, a type of depression caused by low levels of light, seem to react well to a boost of St.-John's-wort, especially when it is combined with lemon balm.

Researchers are also now investigating St.-John's-wort's antiviral potential, including its use as a very promising treatment against HIV infection, Epstein-Barr virus, influenza, herpes, and viral hepatitis infection.

How to Use St.-John's-Wort

St.-John's-wort is often recommended for the treatment of mild to moderate depression. Currently products are standardized to a certain percentage of one of two components: hypericin or hyperforin. The recommended dosage is 900 mg daily, taken in three separate doses of 300 mg each. The positive effects of St.-John's-wort are not immediately evident; it may take 2 to 6 weeks of use before results are noticed.

Standardized St.-John's-wort capsules and tablets are showing up on the shelves of supermarkets and pharmacies as well as in natural-food stores. Tinctures are also often available. In addition, St.-John's-wort infused oil or salve is used to treat external skin conditions. Homeopathic formulations of St.-John's-wort, labeled with the plant's Latin name, *Hypericum perforatum,* are used for the treatment of nerve pain.

ST.-JOHN'S-WORT OIL

This infused oil is wonderful for topical treatment of bruises and sprains.

2–3   **ounces (56–84 g) dried or fresh-wilted St.-John's-wort leaves**
1   **pint (473 ml) olive oil**

1. Put the St.-John's-wort in a jar and add the oil, making sure there are 2 to 3 inches (5–7.5 cm) of oil on top of the herb.

2. Place the jar in a warm, dry spot (such as a sunny windowsill) for 2 weeks. Gently shake the jar every 2 or 3 days.

3. Strain and press the oil from the St.-John's-wort. Let the oil sit until any residual water separates out; then pour off the oil and store it in an airtight container in a cool, dark location, where it will keep for 3 to 6 months.

Safety and Cautions for St.-John's-Wort

When ingested, St.-John's-wort may cause photosensitivity. This side effect was initially observed in animals grazing on large quantities of the wild plant. Since that finding, researchers have questioned whether this effect is replicated in humans and, if so, if it would affect all people or only fair-skinned users. The *PDR for Herbal Medicines* states that photosensitivity in humans is unlikely with the administration of therapeutic dosages. In any case, those taking photosensitizing medications, such as tetracycline, should be careful of sun exposure if supplementing with St.-John's-wort.

A second important caution is for those wanting to treat depression. Depression is not just feeling down or blue; it is a medical condition with possible serious consequences. A depressed person should confer with a professional to get a correct diagnosis, including an evaluation of the severity of symptoms. Do not take St.-John's-wort while taking any other antidepressant, and if you are taking prescription antidepressants, do not abruptly stop their use to switch to St.-John's-wort.

Valerian (*Valeriana officinalis*)

Cats love valerian, maybe for the same reason that most people are repulsed by it — valerian stinks! There are palatable ways to ingest this powerful herbal sedative. Valerian is the premier herb for restless nights and is also a wonderful muscle relaxant, alleviating back pain and menstrual cramps.

Valerian in the Garden

A perennial plant, valerian grows wild in North America and is grown commercially in Europe. It is adored by many gardeners for its good looks and shunned by others because of its fetid smell. Those who like the aroma describe it as a spicy scent reminiscent of the deep woods. The plant grows up to 5 feet (1.5 m) and has long fernlike leaves. The white to pink and lavender flowers are small and grow in branched clusters at the top of the plant. The root of valerian, which has a particularly definitive strong odor, is the part of the plant used medicinally.

Health Benefits

Valerian is the herb of choice for insomnia and stress. It also works well for reducing menstrual cramps, headaches associated with the menstrual cycle, other muscle cramps, and intestinal upsets. The FDA places it on its list of herbs "generally regarded as safe."

German studies have substantiated its benefits as a relaxant without dreaded sedative side effects. Those who take it at night have been rewarded with deep sleep and wake refreshed in the morning. Valerian eliminates the morning-after grogginess associated with chemical tranquilizers. Herbalists recommend valerian as a nonaddictive and non-habit-forming remedy.

Animal studies have indicated that valerian may be helpful in lowering high blood pressure and as an anticonvulsant.

Herbal History

Like many herbal remedies, valerian has a proud history of use. The famous German abbess and herbalist Hildegard von Bingen recommended valerian as a tranquilizer and sleep aid in the twelfth century. Europeans included valerian in formulas to treat conditions ranging from the plague to epilepsy. It was supposedly the hypnotic employed by the Pied Piper of Hamelin to rid the town of rats. Throughout history, it has also been used as a tranquilizer for humans.

How to Use Valerian

The root of the valerian plant is used medicinally. Various preparations are available. The recommended dose of valerian, as with other herbs, depends on the form and brand taken. Many herbalists recommend a dropperful of the tincture in some water at bedtime to benefit from its relaxing qualities. Dr. Andrew Weil, the well-known physician and author, believes that valerian can be especially helpful to those weaning themselves off synthetic sleep aids.

Valerian's primary drawback is its strong, unpleasant odor, often compared to the smell of dirty socks. To overcome this real aesthetic disadvantage, I recommend taking valerian in its more palatable forms, either as a capsule or as a tincture, and not as a tea. Although the strong taste is still evident in the tincture, this form may be chosen for its strength. Combining it with tastier herbs like chamomile, catnip, peppermint, and lemon balm is a good alternative. As a secondary ingredient blended with other, sweeter-scented herbs, valerian can also be used effectively in soothing herbal baths.

VALERIAN TEA

Excerpted from *Rosemary Gladstar's Herbs for Reducing Stress and Anxiety*, by Rosemary Gladstar (Storey Books, 1999).

A hearty, relaxing blend, this tea is one of the better-tasting valerian blends.

½   part dried licorice root
Water
1   part dried valerian root
2   parts dried lemon balm

1. Combine the licorice and water in a large pot. Use approximately 1 cup (237 ml) per teaspoon (5 ml) of herb. Bring to a boil, cover, and simmer for 15 minutes. Remove from heat.

2. Add the valerian and lemon balm. Cover and let steep for 45 minutes.

3. Strain; drink as much and as often as needed.

Safety and Cautions for Valerian

In larger-than-recommended dosages, valerian can cause morning grogginess, nausea, headache, and blurred vision. In a small percentage of users, valerian causes the opposite effect of what is desired — it is stimulating rather than relaxing. These symptoms immediately disappear when the herb is discontinued. Some herbalists assert that long-term valerian use may exacerbate depression.